Belly Fat

BY EMILY HOSKINS

*The Healthy Eating Guide to Lose That
Stubborn Belly Fat - No Exercise
Required*

2nd Edition

Emily Hoskins

Emily Hoskins

Table of Contents

Introduction

Losing weight can take a lot of dedication and hard work in order to see the results that you want. Losing that extra fat that is on your belly can be even more difficult. This is one of the most stubborn areas on the body for keeping that fat. This guidebook is meant to provide you with all of the tips that you need in order to lose the weight on your belly so that you can get the toned and lean body you have always dreamed of.

There is information on what the belly fat diet plan is about, the types of foods that you should eat to melt the belly fat, the foods that you should avoid, and how exercise is able to make the belly fat disappear even more quickly. Use this guidebook to help you to get started in the right direction today.

It also contains information on lifestyle as this is also something to consider when trying to get in shape. You may not know it, but your lifestyle may be the stumbling block that is causing you so much trouble. The reasons are explained and common sense steps are included to help you to get over this aspect. It isn't always what you eat that makes that fat stay. Read through the book and you may even discover you are doing something fundamentally unwise and that stopping that activity in its tracks could help you to get nimble and slim, so that the belly fat drops off.

Did you know that people can do this at any age? They can. Although the metabolism may slow down as you get older, there's no reason to let it get in the way of shaping up. Take a look around you and you will see people who are the same age as you, but who look years younger. You could look like that, but you need to want to and that's the first step in getting that belly fat to melt down into nothing.

I hope you enjoy it

Chapter 1
The Basics

Are you tired of all that extra weight sitting on your belly or hips? Are you tired of not being able to show off your stomach or wear the clothes that you have always wanted because you do not feel like they look good? Then the belly fat diet is the right one for you to try out today.

If you are ready to get that belly fat gone and make the lifestyle changes that are necessary in order to maintain a weight that is healthy, then the belly fat diet plan is the one to try. This is not a crazy fad diet; instead, it is a plan that is going to help you see results for the long term. There are some main principles of this diet that you should keep in mind for the best results. These would include:

- **Eat sufficient food**—it is important that while you are on this diet you do not skip meals. This is just going to make you hungry so when you do eat you will eat too fast and in turn eat too much. This is a mistake made by many. If you are feeling terribly hungry, you tend to grab those foods which give instant gratification without giving real thought to what you are eating. These are the foods which encourage belly fat in the first place. Celebrate your food and be aware of what you are feeding yourself.

Take your time to eat and enjoy the delicious tastes of good foods, putting aside that yen for foods which will only add to your problems.

- **Start eating whole grains**—those white breads that you are eating are simply making you fat. Breads that contain a lot of whole grains are much richer in nutrients and fiber so you will be able to stay full for longer while also preventing any spikes that can happen in your insulin levels. These spikes in insulin are what will trigger the storage of belly fat. Thus, you need to avoid that happening.

- **Being active**—even if you have not started on an exercise routine, purchase a pedometer and make sure that you are getting at least 10,000 steps into your day. This movement is going to stop the belly fat from sticking. There are also fun ways to keep active and these are included in future chapters. Exercise doesn't have to be a chore.

- **Eat fresh farm produce**—one of the best things that you can do for your body is to include eating plenty of fruits and vegetables. These produce have lots of nutrients such as filling fiber and other antioxidants that are going to fight off disease. They are also low in calories so you will not have to worry about gaining a lot of weight from them. Try to make your diet varied so that you have new tastes to look forward to. People see vegetables as being boring, but you really can produce meals that are delicious, using the right types of cooking method and the right kinds of flavorings.

- **Avoid foods that cause inflammation**—these foods are able to trigger the storage of belly fat as well as cause many diseases. Some foods that you should avoid that fit into this category are highly processed foods, trans-fats, saturated fats, and refined carbs. If it's in a packet or a can, read the content. Often, you may think that you are eating healthy food, but will often find that the ingredients of prepared foods are what is causing you inflammation.

- **Eat a health fat each day**—omega-3 fatty acids and monounsaturated fats can help to fight inflammation and belly fat at the same time. These kinds of fats are necessary in order to maintain a body weight that is desirable and they can help you to not get certain diseases. Look in later chapters as this is demonstrated and will show you how to incorporate the omega-3 fatty acids into your diet.

- **Drink 8 cups of water each day**—staying hydrated is important to keeping your energy levels up, can fill you up so that you are not eating as much during your meals, and is a great asset to your metabolism. So make sure that you are getting plenty of water each day. There are other reasons for drinking water. Water helps your body to digest the foods that you eat. Please note that coffee and tea, although made out of water, do not count as part of your daily requirement.

- **Be mindful of your eating**—this is going to take some time. You will need to learn to satisfy the hunger cues of your body in order to get the weight loss to stick around for life. Once you become mindful, you really will enjoy your food more and appreciate taking your time to eat it. Fast foods are not your best friend. They may save time in preparation but they may be knocking years off your life-span.

It is important to keep a balance about your life if you would like to maintain your weight. It is a good idea to follow the 80/20 rule. You should focus about 80 percent of the time on eating foods that are friendly to your belly and will fight inflammation while the other 20 percent you can give yourself some leeway to go off track and splurge. Often people will choose to pick one day where they can have something that is a splurge that is not always on the diet plan. This is a good way to make sure that you stay on the diet because you will be able to look forward to the treat later on.

One way to achieve this is to tell yourself that you can only have that particular treat on a specific day. For example, if you have the family round at weekends, then having one particular dessert that you like won't kill you. Dietary sense isn't about deprivation. It's about learning what's good for the body and what is not. After a while of being sensible about what you eat, you will be able to recognize the messages that your body is trying to give you. Have you ever felt so full that you find your waistline is uncomfortable? We all have, but on a sensible diet made up of the right things, you really will feel better in yourself and will have less tendency to splurge.

Have you ever heard of yo-yo dieting? This is when people go on a specific diet until they reach a certain goal and then immediately go back to their old habits. The problem with this kind of philosophy is that it simply doesn't work. If you deprive your body unduly of foods that you like and then go back to eating them as soon as D-Day arrives, you pile on the weight faster than you would have before you started the diet. It's nonsense and although you may get short term gain, you may be letting yourself in for long term pain.

Carrying excess weight puts a strain on your body. Your heart, your lungs, your mobility all depend upon being fed the right kinds of food. If you fed a car that takes diesel with petrol, it wouldn't work and yet every day, people all over the world feed foods to their bodies which are unhealthy and then wonder why the belly fat is piling up.

The moment you feel unhappy with your body, it's time to realize that only you can make a difference to your future health and by taking this decision to lose that belly fat, you are also taking a decision to improve your health and to show great example to friends and family that will help them to overcome problems of this nature.

You may not realize it, but kids learn by example. At this moment in time, the figures for obesity among children are unacceptably high. These increase the chances of children suffering from diabetes and from heart problems. If you can't do it for you, do it for them. Now is the first day of the rest of your life, and it's time to stop blaming life and take the world by storm. You can do it. There are so many success stories that you could become one of them as well, by following the plan in the following chapters.

Chapter 2
Foods That Burn Belly Fat

Now that you know a little bit more about this diet plan, it is time that you learn which foods you are allowed to eat in order to make the belly fat go away. It is important that you take the time to eat the right kinds of foods if you want to see the results that you want. Here are some of the most important foods that you should include in your day if you want to see the fat melt away.

The first thing that you should try to get into your diet is oatmeal. When you are feeling that morning snack attack coming on, it is usually due to the fact that your blood sugar levels have dipped after eating that sugary breakfast option. It is better to choose an option that is full of fiber such as oatmeal. These foods are able to stay inside your stomach for hours so you will not have to worry about getting that snack in later that day. It is a good idea to watch out for any of the sugary varieties that are available. It is best to choose one that is plain and then sweeten it at home with some berries.

Cereal bars often have a lot of hidden sugar. You need to keep an eye on labels because although they may be marked as being a healthy alternative to eating breakfast, they may actually be causing hunger mid-morning or be responsible for spikes in insulin levels. Thus oats in their natural format are a much better option, even when cooked. Getting back to basics is often a better thing than buying things which purport to be healthy, but which in fact are filled with either sugar or sugar substitutes.

The problem with sugar substitutes is that they are often sweeter than sugar and the sugar spike doesn't last as long as natural sugar. Therefore, your need for the sweeteners increases and you are likely to eat or drink more of the kinds of foods and drinks that contain them because your sugar needs are not being met.

Almonds and nuts can make a great snack if you are looking for something that is tasty and can make the belly fat go away. These kinds of nuts are able to slim down the tummy because they are keeping you full. A study done at Purdue University showed that those who at nuts were able to feel full for a longer tie compared to those who ate rice cakes. It is best to stick to about 24 almonds each day in order to satisfy those hunger pains without overdoing the calories too much. Also, make sure to skip the salted nuts because too much sodium is going to raise your blood pressure. Sodium is responsible for so many problems and unfortunately, the average US diet includes too much. Again, look at labels as often sodium is hidden within prepared foods that you may not even suspect.

Olive oil is a great way to get some of the fat that you need in your diet. While many people worry about eating fat, especially when they are trying to get rid of the fat in their belly, it is important because it is able to control hunger. It is best to choose a monounsaturated variety such as canola or olive oil. These will help to keep your cholesterol levels down while also satisfying any cravings that you have. Make sure to steer away from any hydrogenated vegetable oils. They are going to be loaded with the trans-fats that are unhealthy for you. Olive oil can be used for dressing a salad or even giving a little more flavor to vegetables. In Europe, it is common to use virgin olive oil as this is better than other types. Its taste is good and it's purer.

When you are on the belly fat diet plan, it is a good idea to eat plenty of berries. These are stuffed with the filling fiber that you need in a little package. For example, a cup of raspberries is going to have six grams of fiber in them. You should never use jelly as a substitute for your berries because it is like the junk food in the fruit world. These jellies have a ton of extra sugar and no fiber in them so you are not getting the same health benefits. It is the actual fruit that has the fiber you need and frozen ones may have lost some of the elements you need in your diet. If you can buy berries fresh, then these are always going to be the best bet.

If you want to keep your metabolism going strong, it is a good idea to take in plenty of the important vitamin B12, which can be found in abundance in eggs. According to research done at Louisiana State University, those who at eggs each day for breakfast were able to lose more weight compared to those who ate bagels. Before you start eating eggs it is best to talk with your doctor, especially if you have high cholesterol levels. Remember, there are many ways of cooking eggs and if you really don't want fat in the meal, try boiled or poached eggs as these are delicious and are simple to cook in water.

Legumes and beans are the next food group that you should try to get into your diet. Beans are low in calories while also being full of the fiber and the protein that your body needs in order to lose weight and to tone up. It is a good idea to make dishes that contain a lot of beans such as burritos, instead of using meat, at least once each week. This is going to help you to cut out a lot of saturated fat while increasing the amount of fiber you consume. You should watch out for refried beans though since these are still high in saturated fats. Choose to go with pinto, plain black, and some other varieties for the best results. Be aware that you may need to drink more water when you do increase the amount of beans that you eat, to help your digestion and to help settle down any wind that they may cause.

Fish and lean meats are another choice that you should make. Your body is going to go through more calories when it is digesting proteins compared to fat or carbs. It is best to choose the leanest meats out there so that you are able to get the protein and other nutrients without the extra fat. Turkey is a good option but one of the best is fish. Try to go for options such as salmon and tuna because they are full of the omega-3s that your body needs in order to prevent the belly fat from accumulating. Fresh fish is really good for you and can help you to feel satisfied. It has a lot of goodness and, although it may cost a little more than buying frozen fish, tastes wonderful. Chicken is fine if you stick to eating the white of the meat and avoid eating the skin. Most fast food outlets add flavors to the skin of chicken to make it more delicious, but all of this camouflaging of food is taking away your taste for what's really good for you. It is also quite likely that fast food chicken is fried in the wrong kind of fat.

One meat that you may not have taken much notice of is duck, although perhaps you should. Duck is a very healthy meat to eat. It's great for your immune system and as long as you avoid eating the skin, it's also not that fattening.

Many people who go on a diet feel that carbs are a bad thing and that they should not enjoy them at all. In reality, if you are able to eat the right kinds of carbs, you are going to be getting a lot of the nutrients that your body needs. When you are eating carbs, you should go for the whole grain options so that you can get the fiber that is needed to prevent you from getting hungry. Make sure to watch out for the bread labels. Some of the breads that are labeled with wheat have been stripped of the nutrients and fiber. Make sure to pick the options that are whole grain or 100 percent whole wheat. The trouble is that manufacturers are taking advantage of people liking fast foods and unhealthy breads. Yes, it's easier to eat but it's not the best thing to consider when you have belly fat.

Another food that you are able to enjoy to lose belly fat is peanut butter. This food source is full of niacin, which is going to keep the digestive system on track as well as stopping any belly bloat that you have. It is important to watch out for the portion size that you are enjoying since peanut butter contains a lot of fat. It is a good idea to limit the consumption to two tablespoons or less a day. Also, pick out the options of peanut butter that are all natural because they are not going to contain extra sugar.

Green vegetables are full of the minerals and vitamins that your body needs in order to stay strong in addition to making your waist line smaller. There are lots of different vegetables that will fit into this category such as broccoli and spinach and they are loaded with lots of fiber as well as only a few calories. You should try and create a salad with these kinds of vegetables before you eat so that you are feeling fuller even with the smaller portions. Try to fill up with some spinach, arugula, or romaine lettuce rather than iceberg lettuce since it does not have much fiber.

Dairy is not something that you should be avoiding when you go on one of these diets. The calcium is able to help break down the fat in your body and in some cases it is able to prevent fat from forming in the first place. You should make sure and pick the fat free or low fat versions so that you are not taking in too many calories. Be careful here because manufacturers know what's tasty and they may be supplementing the taste with aspartame. That's not the healthiest of alternatives. If you choose low fat plain yogurts you can always add a small spoon of brown sugar and do your body less harm.

Avocados are a great source of fiber and monounsaturated fats, both of which are going to be great at keeping you full for longer. In fact, you are going to be able to get up to 17 grams of fiber from each avocado. If you are able to eat about half a cup each day you will be able to stave off any hunger pains that you have.

Iced or green tea is a good option because they are full of the antioxidants that you will need in order to speed up your metabolism. The faster that you can get your metabolism to go, the more fat you will be using up. According to studies, those who drink this kind of tea are shown to burn up an extra 266 calories each day compared to those who do not drink tea. You should try and avoid the bottled teas because they are short on the slimming nutrients that you need as well as having a lot of extra calories in them. Instead, you should steep a bag of tea in some hat water for a few minutes, cool down with a few ice cubes, and then enjoy. You should do this four times a day for the best results.

Parmigiano-Reggiano cheese is a low calorie snack that includes the calcium that you need in order to activate the hormones for burning fat in the body according to research done at the University of Wisconsin. Plus, the high content of protein, much more than what is found in other dairy products, you will be able to stay full for a longer period of time. The best way to get this food is to grate an ounce of it over your soups and enjoy.

Cannellini beans are a great starch that has a type of fiber that is difficult to digest so these are going to cause a punch. If your stomach is taking longer to digest something, you are going to feel fuller for longer and you will be burning more weight at the same time. The slower digestion is going to work in order to have the body doing more, which is going to burn up more calories just to burn the calories. You will be able to battle up the belly fat with about half a cup each day.

Chapter 3
Foods to Avoid

Not only are you going to be having to watch the foods that you should eat in order to lose your belly fat, it is also important that you make sure to avoid certain food products. These products are known to cause more fat to be in the body and can increase the amount of body fat that is in your belly. This chapter is going to talk about some of the foods that you should avoid if you are serious about getting rid of the belly fat that is around your middle.

The first thing that you are going to need to cut out of your diet is soda. Not only is soda very unhealthy for your body, but it is known to increase the amount of fat that you have around your belly. This product is full of empty calories that will add excess weight to your body. You are also going to be adding in a lot of sugar to your body; this kind of sugar is going to come from the high fructose corn sugar as well as from other additives that are in the soda to give it its flavoring and color. Your body is going to have a difficult time in burning all of this sugar, especially once it gets to the abdomen. The high fructose corn syrup is enough to make you obese, especially when it comes to your middle. Many people will think that consuming diet sodas is a better option, but these options are going to contain other artificial sweeteners that will contribute to bad health. It is often best to just drink water in order to lose the belly fat.

Everyone likes to have a dessert after their main meal and it is often the most popular part of the meal. But it is important to realize that these desserts are full of a lot of extra calories that are going to ruin your diet. Even if the dessert is one that is low in calories and in fat, you should make sure to only eat them in moderation so that you are not throwing the whole diet out the window. Most of the desserts that you will pick have some refined sugars that will lead to gaining of weight in your body. It is best to eat some form of fruit rather than candies, cookies, and cakes. This does not mean that you cannot have a dessert every once in a while; you just need to make sure to enjoy it in moderation and not have it too often.

When you are trying to get rid of the fat that is around your middle, it is best that you avoid fast food completely. This is the worst kind of food for your belly because the fries, shakes, and burgers are going to have a lot of carbs, fat, and calories that your body is not going to need so it will end up storing them in your body. None of these things are nutritious and they will just lead to more of a belly. In addition, the foods that you eat from fast food restaurants are cooked in fatty oils; these are the kind of oils that are known to contribute to obesity.

Whole fat milks are not good for your midsection. Sure, you will still be able to get all of the calcium as well as other nutrients from drinking this milk, but you will also be consuming more fat content in the process. When you are an adult, it is usually not necessary to drink whole milk unless you are dealing with issues of not gaining weight. You will be able to drink skimmed or another low fat option and still get the same nutrients without worrying about the extra fat. This can help you to maintain the healthy weight that you want without the extra stuff. Again, watch out for what's in the milk. If you buy low fat milk, often the taste is added to by manufacturers to make the milk more palatable.

Potato chips are another snack that could be adding in to the belly fat. Most of the brands that you can buy will be cooked in hydrogenated oils which is a type of trans-fat. This is a type of fat that is known to increase your cholesterol levels and eventually lead to increased weight and heart disease. Even if you choose a potato chip that is cooked in other oils, there are still going to be high amounts of oil. There are some other options, such as low fat and baked potato chips, that are on the market and can be a better choice if you need to wean yourself off the potato chips. But it is still important that you are aware of the calorie counts that are in these chips because the higher calories can still increase your belly fat.

Pancakes and other breakfast foods that you will need to avoid if you want to get rid of the stubborn belly fat. While these might be delicious to have right away in the morning, they are going to contain a lot of fat and calories that are really harmful to your belly. Eating this food can be even worse when you are topping it with the syrup. Even pancakes that are considered light can add to the amount of fat that you have in your belly. It is better to avoid the pancakes and enjoy some whole wheat waffles instead in the morning.

These are all some of the foods that you will need to avoid if you would like to see a difference in your waistline. With this kind of diet plan it is important that you watch not only the foods that you are taking in but you will also need to make sure that you are avoiding any of the foods that were listed above. Also, keep all of the other processed and sugary foods that you love out of your diet because they will not offer much nutritional value, can make you hungry quickly, will mess with your blood sugar levels, and are really high in fats and calories.

Remember, when you are eating to be conscious of what you eat and listen to your body. It will tell you when you have had enough. There's no obligation for you to take more food than your body needs and, in fact, loading your plate down with food has probably had a lot to do with the increase in your belly size. Cut down the portions and enjoy what you have without that horrible feeling of discomfort after each meal.

Chapter 4
Bad Habits In Lifestyle

Although you may not be aware of it, you may have acquired habits over the course of your life which are not only detrimental to your health, but which may actually be making the belly fat worse. One of these is that you may not be going to the toilet enough. That may sound a little crazy but do you spend a lot of time constipated? It's important enough to consider as part of your lifestyle if you get chronic constipation.

There are a number of reasons for this and although people blame their digestive system, they may not be helping because they eat on the go, or they eat too fast. One of the things that was mentioned in a previous chapter was taking the time to be mindful of the food that you eat. If you take a look around a restaurant at how people eat, you will instantly recognize those who don't take their time and many of them will have belly fat.

Digestion needs your help. You need to chew your food more and to take your time when eating. Being mindful is not just being aware of what you are eating, but being aware of the eating process as well. If you simply wait until you are constipated and then take a pill, that food is staying in your belly and it fermenting. This means that it is creating gases that shouldn't be there.

You need to get into the habit of taking sufficient time to eat and also of drinking plenty of water. People who lack drinking water in their diet will find that they can suffer bad cramps because the water is needed to stop your body from dehydrating. Busy lives often mean that people eat quickly, they don't drink enough water and as a consequence tend to get constipated. Some people can go several days without a bowel movement and it's healthy to make the effort every day to let that waste out.

If you are one of those who has never paid much attention to chewing your food sufficiently, then chances are that you also miss out on being regular and this isn't good for the belly area of your body.

To overcome this, be conscious of what you are eating. Don't swallow until the food is chewed and enjoy what you eat. Often rushed lives mean that food goes down too fast and that's a real mistake where body fat is concerned.

Think this isn't a serious problem?

According to Livestrong.com, who have collated information on constipation, more than 4 million

American people suffer from constipation and bloating and that over half of these will visit their doctor for help to overcome the problem.

If you deprive yourself of carbs, what happens is that the body takes the carbs it needs from the storage within your body. While you may think this is what you want your body to do, it is actually harming you because it takes natural liquid from your body that you may not be replacing with water. The vicious circle of constipation and taking laxatives makes your bowels less effective at getting rid of waste. This, in turn, means that your body becomes too dependent upon laxatives and doesn't make the effort itself to go regularly. Thus, you do need carbohydrates in sensible amounts, but you also need water to help your digestion and to make the foods that you eat easier to digest.

Coffee

Yes, we are all guilty of loving a cup of coffee, but did you know that for every cup that you drink, you actually urinate almost three times as much liquid as you take in. This is why we advised that you can't use coffee as a substitute for water. It dehydrates the body and can become another vicious circle, where your body tells you that you need another drink. The natural drink to reach out for is coffee, which will dehydrate you even further.

It's important when you want to lose belly fat that you recognize that water is an essential part of your diet. It's vital. If you are having problems with your digestion and notice changes in your bowel movements or sudden weight loss, then of course, you should go to the doctor. If, however you have read the above and are guilty of one or more of the following, you need to change your lifestyle:

> - Eating too quickly – not chewing food enough
> - Not drinking enough water
> - Depending on medications to pass stools

All of these are signs that you need to take more time eating. You also need to drink more water and take the time to sit leisurely on the toilet and let your body do the work it needs to do to keep you healthy and keep your belly fat at bay.

Chapter 5
The Importance Of Sleep

Often people who have busy lives don't get the sleep that they need, or feel tired for much of the time. The quality of your sleep matters as well as the duration. Some people need less than others, but you may just be going to bed with too much undigested food in your system and may need to change a few habits to help you to get sufficient rest.

If you are lethargic, this is a good sign that you're not getting the rest you need and believe it or not, during the sleep cycle, your body is healing and recovering from the day before, making it ready for the day to come. There are many other things that happen during sleep but if you are trying to lose belly fat, you need that extra energy the next day, so that you can function at an optimal level and be more inclined to exercise, even if that just means going for a walk.

Many obese people don't get enough sleep or go the other way and become too lazy, staying in bed for far too long. Striking the balance is essential to good health. The danger is that people who are inactive encourage the build-up of visceral fat in the belly region and that's deep fat that is harmful to areas of the body such as your heart or your lungs. Thus, it's important to be active, but if you are sleepy, that's hard.

So how much sleep is healthy?

There have been studies into this aspect of life and although some people believe that 8 hours is correct, they may be doing themselves a disservice. Between six and seven hours a night is enough, but it should be quality sleep.

How does that affect the belly region?

If you sleep well, you are much more energetic the next day and are able to use that energy to give yourself a head start when it comes to being active. The vision that people think of when they associate thoughts with obesity is inactivity and that's the same for belly fat too. If you are constantly inactive, don't get enough sleep and eat all the wrong things, you don't stand a chance of losing belly fat.

If you sleep well and don't allow stresses to keep you out of bed, you will give yourself a better start the next day. If you have eaten too close to bedtime, and usually these are snacks, you can't get the quality sleep that you need and thus, you wake tired and spend much of the next day feeling like you have no energy.

Food before bedtime

There are all sorts of myths about how soon before bedtime you should stop eating. You do need your evening meal, so don't skimp on that, but the area when you really put your belly fat at risk of increasing is when you eat high calorie, high sugar or fat foods as a snack before bedtime. The kind of snacks that should be avoided at this time of day are:

> ➢ Ice cream – substitute with fruit sorbet if you like or fresh fruit such as a banana.
> ➢ Potato chips – These are unhealthy anyway, but before bedtime, they don't digest easily.
> ➢ Popcorn – this is only unhealthy if coated. If you eat fresh popped popcorn, it's not going to harm you, but you may take time to fully digest it.

Eat light foods before bedtime and if you are puckish, a few nuts or raisons are much better for you that heavy foods.

Trouble sleeping?

If you are experiencing trouble sleeping, perhaps you are not preparing yourself for sleep. The bedroom should be a place where you can completely relax. If you use the breathing exercises in the next chapter at bedtime, these will help you to wind down and to forget the stresses of the day. Try to avoid television programs that are too active just before you go to bed and start thinking of your bedroom as being a place where you can wind down.

If you practice the breathing exercises, these will help your stress levels and you will find that they may also help you to get sufficient sleep to wake up fresh and ready for action the next day.

Sleep is important to you, regardless of whether you want to lose weight or not. In the case of belly fat, it gives your body time to recharge and that's vital to successfully losing that fat. A tired and stressed body won't respond as well to the need to exercise. Thus, if you can get a good night's sleep, you will be able to exercise more the following day, thus helping you to lose that belly fat.

Chapter 6
Breathing Exercises to Help You Lose Belly Fat

You may not be aware of it but certain breathing exercises can help you to lose that belly fat, as long as they are able to work hand in hand with sensible diet and a reasonable amount of exercise. These can be done before going to bed and as they take a little time to perform, allow yourself that time before bedtime because it will be worth it. Stress plays a lot in whether people lose belly fat and those who are able to let go of that stress using breathing exercises will benefit enormously.

It may be handy to have an exercise mat for these exercises, since this supports the body in the right position for the lying down exercises and is better than a sprung mattress which affects the way that your posture is set while lying down.

Exercise 1 – Tummy toning

Lie on your back with your hands by your sides and your legs bent, feet flat on the floor. This is a comfortable position for those with extra belly fat. It's also a great position to feel the belly area being worked. Pull your tummy in as far as you are able and hold it to the count of 10 seconds. Let the air out of your body slowly and if you want to use a hand on the abdomen area to feel yourself pulling it in before making that ten second count, then that works as well. This is an exercise that you can perform at any time of the day, whether standing, sitting or lying down, but it helps to familiarize yourself with that feeling of the tummy being pulled in entirely in this lying down position. If you practice this during your working day, no one will notice but you and long term, you really will find it makes a difference.

Exercise 2 – The hard pull

This is another exercise that you can do at night, when you haven't just eaten. You need to kneel on the mat and lean forward, keeping your back curved upward and leaning down with your hands on the mat in front of you. This position helps you to get maximum pull on your belly area. Breathe in as normal, and then as you breathe out to the count of ten seconds, pull your tummy in as far as you are able. Hold you tummy in that position and count to ten. This exercise can be repeated up to 10 times in a day.

Exercise 3 – Breathing from the Abdomen

You may not be aware of it, but the breathing used in this exercise helps you in many ways. It helps to get rid of stress and it helps your body to feel more aligned. It also helps your abdominal region to work a little bit which contributes to loss of belly fat.

Lie down on your bed and support your head with a pillow. If you are not too comfortable with your back straight, you can bend your knees and place your feet on the bed. Breathe in through the mouth to the count of ten. When you breathe out, instead of moving your chest, be aware of the breathing coming from your abdominal area. Place your hand on your tummy. As you breathe out, your tummy should rise, rather than the chest area.

If you need to place your hand on your chest you can do this, but don't do it to the extent that it hurts. This helps your posture and thus will help to align your belly fat area. It helps the muscles in this area to work harder and also aligns the spine. Take it easily. If it's a little hard at first, stop if you feel strain and then try again, but be aware of your body when you do the exercise. If it needs to stop, stop. The idea is not to cause pain, but to work the abdominal area of the body so that your digestion is better and you feel fitter and stronger.

Breathing through the Mouth

Although you may think that it's not a good thing to breathe through the mouth, it will help you to calm your stress levels so is a great exercise for just before you go to bed. Lying on your back in bed, breathe in through the mouth to a count of 4 and then exhale through the mouth to the count of 6. You only need to do this a couple of times at night and can increase your exercises or decrease it when you like. The idea is to help you to sleep better, so it's ideal for bedtime.

There is one more exercise I would like to introduce but this isn't suitable for bedtime. You need to practice this in the morning as it energizes and that's not what you need just before you go to bed.

Sit in an upright position which is comfortable. A hard chair is suitable. Place your hands on your belly. As you inhale, be aware that you are taking in as much air as you can comfortably. Then press on your tummy and tense the muscles in that area while you exhale. This is a great exercise and you will get better at it with practice. Doing this, three times in the morning before you face your day will really help you to become energized and focused on life and that will help you with your belly fat challenge.

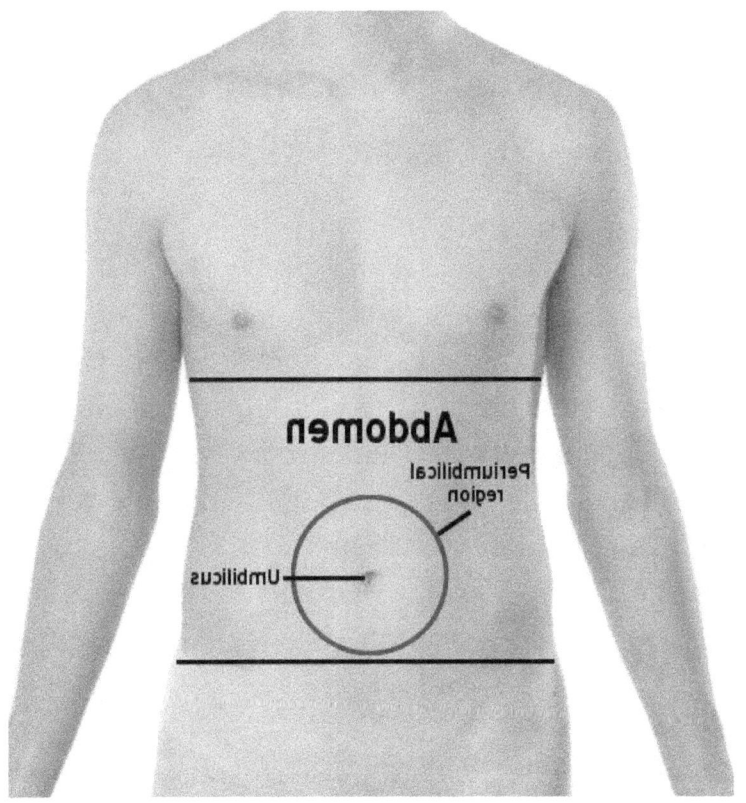

Remember, your abdomen is where you feel pressure when doing these exercises.

Chapter 7
Having Some Fun Losing Your Belly Fat

You may think that losing that belly fat has to include work and change to your diet and lifestyle, but this can include fun as well. There are several ways that you can incorporate fun into your exercise routine. These will all help you to digest your food in a more efficient way and also help all that excess fat to go away. Do use sense when you use these exercises. Just after a meal is not the ideal time. In the middle of the afternoon or even in the evening before you meal or on a weekend morning, let's show you how to exercise and have fun at the same time.

Walking the dog

This may not feel like it's going to provide much fun but it can if you make it something that you enjoy sharing with family, or if you can set yourself some kind of goal, like arriving at a friend's house or taking the dog to the shop three blocks away. That dog is your reason to exercise. It needs you to take it out for its needs and a pet owner is much more likely to enjoy the walk and not see it as actual exercise. It helps you to get grounded and to have a responsibility to the animal but it can be fun too. Take the dog into the park and play catch with it. Make your pet your friend because walking with the dog can help your digestive system and can also knock off many of the excess calories at the same time.

More fun

There is a dance routine at the moment called Zumba. Most of the people you see in the videos on YouTube are dressed in leotards and lithe and lovely, so that's probably put you off going to a class. If you have belly fat, you feel out of place with all these young people. However, doing Zumba is something you can do privately and make it more enjoyable too.

If you are unfit, you need to prepare for a session. You will need a video on YouTube to accompany your dance routine, which will be done in the comfort of your own home. Think of this as your switch off time. This is your fun and believe me, it really is fun. You need to be dressed in comfortable clothing and be somewhere where you won't be disturbed.

Warming up

Before you do any vigorous exercise at all, you need to limber up. That means shaking your hands, your arms, your legs, just to get the ligaments moving before you put extra stress on them.

Now, switch on the video and let your hair down. It doesn't matter how badly you dance. Imitate the dancers on the screen and have a ball. There was a scene in Ally McBeal where Ally jumped up and down on her bed doing a happy dance to get away from the stresses of life. All you are doing when you are dancing is having fun, burning up calories and giving yourself a little time on your own to feel young again. It doesn't matter what age you are or how badly you dance. It's the rhythm of the music and the shaking of your body to that music that helps to build up your metabolism so that you lose weight.

If you can do this a couple of times a week, you will energize the body. Don't go straight for food after your session. If you need anything at all, take a bottle of mineral water with you into the room where you want to exercise and drink that. Then, when the exercise is finished, a few nuts or raisons will be a good snack to reward yourself for your efforts.

If you think about how kids perceive reading, some will really enjoy it and see it as a step into another world. Others, who have been punished by being forced to read will hate reading and see it as punishment regardless of how much adventure is found with the pages of a book. It's a chore, so they don't do it. In the same way, exercise is perceived as punishment and sometimes it really doesn't have to be. It can be fun as well and you can reap all of the benefits by simply strutting your stuff with Zumba dancing. Dancing is much more likely to be associated with fun because it's a social pastime and thus not thought of in the same way as traditional exercise.

The more you dance, the more you perform the breathing exercises in the last chapter and the more you are aware of your diet, the more likely you are to lose that belly fat.

Zumba is all about letting go of all those pent up emotions. It's about movement and rhythm and it's about exercising each of the parts of the body without even being aware that you are exercising. Now, how cool is that?

This system of dance has no real rules. It means that all of the dance moves are up to you. If you can't stretch, you simply do what you can. You don't take yourself beyond your capabilities, but you let the music guide you into movements that really are fun to do.

If you want to help kids conquer their belly fat or to prevent them from becoming obese, then this is something you could involve them in as well, making it a family fun exercise. However, if you are embarrassed about not being able to dance very well, don't worry. Do the exercise alone.

The fact that you are exercising helps to speed up your metabolism and makes you more able to cope with digesting your food, and more likely to continue in an energetic way through the day that lies ahead.

The first couple of times you do this, you may feel tired after the session, but persist with it and you really will find hidden energy you didn't know you had.

Chapter 8
Exercises to Reduce Belly Fat

If you really want to see some difference in your belly fat, eating is an important part of the process. For those who are able to follow some of the guidelines that were listed above, it can become really easy to see some of the weight loss around the belly that you want. But with this kind of diet plan, the foods that you eat and avoid are not going to be enough in order to see the final results. You are going to need to include some kind of exercise into the mix in order to get the final results. Ok so I know the subtitle of this book has the words "No exercise required", whilst this is true (check out the Bonus section at the end of the book) you can really push through that final barrier to get the flat stomach you've always dreamed of.

Most people think that they need to do a lot of torso twists and crunches in order to get rid of all the excess fat that they have around their lower belly. But this is not always the reality. The most important thing that you can do in order to get rid of that excess belly wait is to get off the mat and then move around as much as possible. Ab exercises can be a great way to build up the muscles that are in that area of the body as well as tone them up, but they are not going to do much for the fat tissue that is there. Instead, you are going to need to do some different exercises that will burn up even more calories. This chapter is going to focus on some of the different exercises that you can do in order to get that belly fat off and look and feel the very best that you can.

The first thing that you need to do is concentrate on targeting the lower belly. This is important because it is going to help you lose your overall body fat. It is not possible to just lose the weight that is around your body, but if you are trying to lose body fat all over the body than you will be able to also lose some around your midsection. Your body is going to be the one that decides where the fat is going to break down. However, as the amount of your total body fat begins to decrease, you will be able to see changes that are present all over the body, even in the stomach. You are not going to be able to do any exercises that will specifically target the lower belly in terms of the fat loss, although they will help with toning up the muscle that is there. Therefore, if you are looking to get rid of the belly fat that is in the way, you will need to do different types of exercises that are meant for fat loss in the whole body.

Now you need to concentrate on how you will be able to lower your body fat in your whole body. This will include doing things like eating a diet that has low calories and fat while also participating in a workout program that will include both strength and cardio training. This is what is going to help you to lose fat because you will start to create a caloric deficit in the body. What this all means is that when you are burning more calories than you are consuming, you are creating a deficit. It is a good idea to create a deficit of between 300 to 500 calories using both exercise as well as decreasing your caloric intake in order to get this deficit. Cardio exercise is a great option to use to burn up the calories and lose the fat. Strength training is going to help develop lean tissue which can sped up the metabolic rate while increasing the amount of calories that you are able to lose during the day.

Firstly, we are going to talk about cardio exercise and what it is able to do in order to help you feel better and lose that stubborn belly fat that you want to get rid of. According to the American Council on exercise, cardio excrcises such as aerobic dancing, basketball, swimming, and running are the best and most efficient to helping you burn up calories and helping you to lose the fat that you want. The number of calories that can be burned will depend on your current weight. For example, a person who weigh 180 pounds will be able to burn around 17 calories for each minute of running that they do and 11.6 for each minute of swimming, 11.3 for each minute of playing basketball, and then 11.1 for each minute that they are dancing aerobically. This is going to vary depending on how big of a person you are. It is recommended that you try to get at least 30 to 50 minutes of some form of cardio activity on most days of the week. It is also a good thing to remember that you are not required to complete a long workout all at once. It is effective to split up the workout into shorter workouts if you do not have 60 minutes to spend on a workout. This means that you could split up the workout into 10 to 15 minutes periods throughout the day and you will be able to get the same benefits of doing it all at once.

While there are a lot of great benefits that you are able to get from doing a good cardio workout during the week, it is important that you take the time to do some weight or strength training as well. Many people are going to skip this activity because they do not feel like they are burning a lot of calories while they are working out. This might be true as lifting up a weight is not going to be that efficient during the workout for burning up the calories that you want, but once you are done it is going to help you increase your calories while you are resting. The toned muscle that you are forming is going to waste a lot more calories and fat even when it is at rest, compared to the fat that is just sitting there. It is a good idea to participate in some type of strength training exercise at least two or three days each week, making sure to have a two day break between each of your workouts.

According to the American Council on Exercise, it is recommended that you complete at least one or two sets that contain 15 repetitions in order to see the fat loss that you want. In addition, if you want to spend your time working towards your ab muscles in specific in order to make them more defined, you should make sure that the strength training workouts that you try to incorporate ab exercises as well. If you are looking for some exercises that are going to be effective for your abs you should try out crunches on top of an exercise ball, straight leg crunch, and bicycle crunch.

Exercise is an important part of your whole weight loss goals. You will not be able to see the changes that you want in your belly fat if you are not able to add in a great exercise program as well. Remember that these exercises, in conjunction with fun exercise such as Zumba and breathing exercises which target the belly area will all help you to lose that belly fat. It took a long time to build it up but it won't take as long to get rid of it if you are prepared to take a little bit of responsibility for it and work toward losing it using these methods.

It's very easy to sit on your laurels and decide to do nothing. Your body is sluggish already and with time will get more sluggish. The fact that you bought this book tells me that you know it's a problem and that you want to find solutions. That should always be in your mind when you eat, exercise, relax or change your lifestyle. The hardest part is keeping the body adequately hydrated and I cannot emphasize enough the importance of water.

Drink plenty before and after your exercise sessions.

Chapter 9
Posture

While you may not think that posture has anything to do with belly fat, it does. Look at the way that you stand and the way that you sit because these elements are all important to the way that your body appears. In a before and after shot on slimming websites, a simple change of stance can make a model look much slimmer than she actually is or much fatter than she is and that's what advertisers depend upon to get you hooked on products to help you lose belly fat. They purport to burn that fat. Look closely at the photographs. There is no magical cure and no matter what the adverts say, it is the posture that makes you believe it may be a viable alternative. The models look like they lost weight.

I saw a program recently where they showed how these different before and after images are taken. Different posture, different light and the angle of the camera make all the difference to what you see on the page. Look closely because the pictures are trying to kid you.

Now, if a photograph can do this, then this must mean that your own posture can make you look a certain way. When you stand with a constant slouch, your shoulders get rounded and after a while this roundness can become part of who you are.

You may remember your parents telling you to sit straight at the table. They had good reason to request that because at the time, your body was growing and developing and they feared that you may develop bad habits that would kick you later in your life.

As time has gone by, you have continued to have posture problems – not because you don't care but perhaps because the couch got too soft. Look at your normal sitting position on a couch. I am sitting on one as I write this and the thing that I noticed the most is that my belly area is sticking out. When I move to a chair which has firm upholstery, this is different and my back is straighter, my tummy tucked in.

With the breathing exercises that were shown in a previous chapter, these can be done while you sit, holding in the belly area, but you can't do it very well if your posture is already slouched and your tummy pushed out by the position in which you are seated.

Be aware of your posture. If there are positions which make your belly area seem bigger then you need to change position and breathe in. Then as you breathe out, pull in your belly to the whole exhalation.

This is something that you can do at any time of day and will help you to get into the habit of making your body as straight as possible and keeping your posture in an acceptable position. The image below shows the seating position which is correct on the right hand side. Notice how straight the back is.

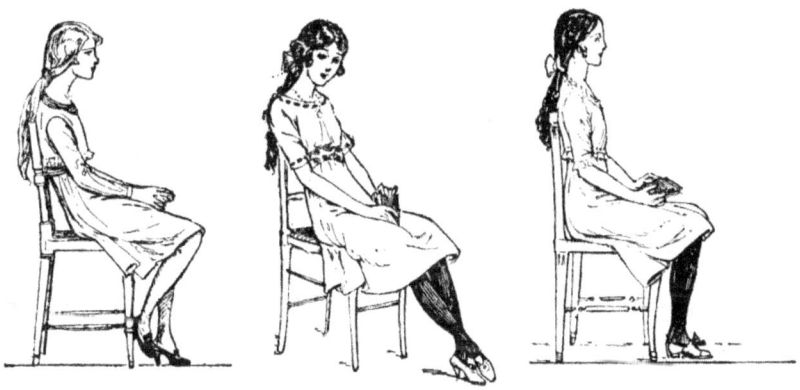

Many people slouch over desks and don't give much regard to how they sit or the position of the spine. In the first image, imagine this in a soft sofa and the abdomen and belly area are pushed out into an unnatural position, putting pressure onto the spine. The second position isn't much better. At least in the first position, the legs are helping to take some of the strain. In the second position, the area which is vulnerable is the lower back and the position also pushes the abdomen forward.

Be conscious of your posture at all times. Learning to breathe correctly and to pull in that belly fat area will help you to lose the weight that you want to lose so that your natural instinct will always be to respect the position of your spine. Once you do, you will find that losing that fat will become a natural extension to your lifestyle and the respect you give to your body.

Conclusion

Losing the fat around your belly can be a challenge. It likes to stick there and you are going to have to take some time and work in order to force it to leave. This book is full of the information that you need in order to get started on the belly fat diet plan so that you can make that stomach go away! Remember, at the end of the day, it is up to you how fast that belly fat goes. Change your eating habits. Substitute butter for Omega Spread, cut down to skimmed milk, be aware of your sugar intake and follow the advice given in the previous chapters about exercise, posture and diet.

As a final note I think it's important to say that everyone has a different body shape to the next person and there is real danger in comparing your body with someone else. Your goal should be to have the healthiest and slimmest version of you that you can achieve. You should aim for the best you! Avoid aiming for the bikini model stomach or the glamour model on the front of your much loved (more than likely heavily photo-shopped) fashion magazine. Just aim for a better you. Take the steps listed in this book, eat well, live an active healthy lifestyle and enjoy your transformation as you say goodbye to that excess, stubborn belly fat!

You can do it and, in fact, you are the only one who can. The example that you set for your kids and for your friends may lead to them wanting to follow the same route. With obesity figures so high throughout the United States, taking this stand against belly fat is your way forward to a healthier life. That belly fat may not yet be dangerous but it can become dangerous when left unchecked. Your life is worth so much more than all of the treats you ate to get you to this stage. Your life is worth the lifestyle changes suggested and you really can look younger and fitter once your lifestyle takes account of your body's needs.

Be aware that crash diets don't work. Be aware that half-hearted exercise doesn't work. Be very aware that the tips and tricks shown in this book have been proven to work time and time again. The food values are well known ones and you probably know what you eat that's bad for you. Remember, you don't have to totally deprive yourself of good things. You merely need to limit these to sensible proportions. The change that you make in your diet, your sleep habits and your exercise routine can add years to your life and that's got to be life-changing.

The best thing of all about losing that belly fat is the comfort that you feel when you wear clothing that looks great. You don't feel like your breathing is impaired. You don't get as much pain and you certainly don't have to obsess about wearing clothing that camouflages the area of your body you know you can do something about. That's when you know you are on the right track. Do it for yourself and be proud of your achievement because with a slim waistline and abdomen area, you really do feel great. You feel less bloated, less uncomfortable and much more able to face the day. You sleep better, you eat better and your body will thank you for all the effort that you have put into losing that belly fat.

If you look at TV programs about weight loss, some of these suggest that surgery is the answer. It's worthwhile thinking about this. In a recent study in the United Kingdom, where limitations are put on who can have surgery for obesity, people were actually putting on weight intentionally to get that surgery. Some even risked their lives for it when the answer lay in their hands all of the time. This book tells you everything that you need to know about losing that belly fat and the belly fat really is the worst kind of fat. Once this goes, the rest of the body seems to be able to function in a more efficient way, meaning that you feel great, look good and can congratulate yourself for taking your responsibility to your body seriously.

Preview of My Other Books

If you are interested in improving your health then you may also be interested in some of my other Amazon Top Ranking books.

Here's a list of a few that you may be interested in checking out.

Gluten-Free: *The Healthy Lifestyle Guide to Gluten-Free Diets*

Sugar Free: *9 Life Changing Reasons To Follow A Sugar Free Diet: The Healthy Lifestyle Guide To Sugar Free Diets.*

Vegan Diet for Beginners - *20 Easy & Delicious Vegan Recipes for Healthy Living*

Smoothies: 14 Nutrient-Packed Smoothies to Help You Detox, Lose Weight and Feel Fantastic

Paleo Diet for Beginners: *Quick And Easy Paleo Recipes To Help You Lose Weight Fast - Easy And Delicious*

Or for some awesome insights on how to live a more confident, relaxed life then check out these:

Self-Esteem For Women*: The Ultimate Women's Guide to Loving Yourself and Building High Self-Esteem*

Meditation For Beginners *- Deep Relaxation Techniques For Long Lasting Peace and Happiness*

Emily Hoskins